Pranayama

The Vedic Science of Breath

14 Ultimate Breathing
Techniques
to Calm Your Mind, Relieve Stress
and Heal Your Body

Advait

Disclaimer and FTC Notice

Pranayama: The Vedic Science of Breath
Copyright © 2017, Advait. All rights reserved.

ISBN 10: 1976443490
ISBN 13: 978-1976443497

The intent of the author is only to offer information of a general nature to help you in your quest for emotional, spiritual and physical well being. In the event you use any of the information in this book for yourself, which is your constitutional right, the author and the publisher assume no responsibility for your actions.

Under no circumstances will any legal responsibility or blame be held against the publisher for any reparation, damages, or monetary loss due to the information herein, either directly or indirectly. The information herein is offered for informational purposes solely, and is universal as so. The presentation of the information is without contract or any type of guarantee assurance.

Adherence to all applicable laws and regulations, including international, federal, state, and local governing professional licensing, business practices, advertising, and all other aspects of doing business in the US, Canada, or any other jurisdiction is the sole responsibility of the purchaser or reader.

Neither the author nor the publisher assumes any responsibility or liability whatsoever on the behalf of the purchaser or reader of these materials.

Any perceived slight of any individual or organization is purely unintentional.

Contents

Pranayama

A Brief History of Yoga

Before starting let's look back at where it all began.

To tell you the truth.... No one knows!!

The foundation of Yoga as a science is attributed to *Maharshi Patanjali* who lived in India in the 3rd Century B.C.

But, archeological excavations in the Indus Valley civilization sites have unearthed sculptures and idols depicting various Asanas (physical exercise positions) suggested in Yoga and these idols date back to around 3000 years B.C.

Also, information about various aspects of Yoga can be found in Vedic texts like; Shwetashwatrupanishad,

Chaandogyopanishad,

Kaushitki Upanishad,

Maitri Upanishad etc.

This information was scattered all over and Maharshi Patanjali, compiled these nuggets into a streamlined and strict science of Yoga or should I say he compiled this scattered information into a way of life called *Yoga* through his work 'Paatanjal YogaSutra'

After Maharshi Patanjali, Maharshi Swatwaram wrote 'Hatapradipika' (meaning - One Which Illuminates the Path of Hatha Yoga , i.e. the physical aspect of Yoga) in the 13th Century A.D.

And, Maharshi Gherand wrote 'Gherandsanhita' around the same time.

Almost all the Yoga methodologies practiced world-over today regard Maharshi Patanjali's work as their reference.

Introduction

The Vedic Science of Breath

Pranayama is considered of paramount importance in Yoga.

The word Pranayama is made of two basic Sanskrit words-

Pran (पूराण) = Life or Universal Life Energy.

Ayam (आयाम) = to Extend and Elongate.

Thus Pranayama means 'an exercise which is to be performed if you want to extend your life'.

Pranayama is the fuel of life...

Here is an interesting analogy-

You are familiar with the existence of the seven (7) chakras along the spine,

which are considered as the energy points sustaining life and health.

Advait

If these Chakras are the rotating wind mills which produce energy to sustain life,

then prana is the essential wind energy which makes the hands of a wind mill rotate, to produce that energy.

When we breathe in we take in the essential oxygen along with the all-pervading Prana.

[And when we breath out we push out the expended energy and toxins out of our body.]

Ayurveda calls our digestion as 'Jathar Agni' literally meaning 'digestive fire', it compares our digestive process with a 'Yadnya' - A holy Pyre, where things are offered to the gods.

And the 'Prana' we take in, is the fuel for this holy Yadnya.

When we practice Pranayama, we regulate and streamline the process of drawing in the universal life force and thus enhancing our health and longevity.

This is the metaphysical Prana aspect of it.

Now let us look at the physical significance, but for that I first need to tell you about our bodies' digestive and excretory mechanism.

We consume food, which is broken down into small pieces by our teeth and is added primary digestive enzymes from the saliva in our mouth.

It then passes into our stomach, where it is churned and more gastric juices are added to it to induce breakdown of the food consumed.

This mixture then passes through our intestines, whose walls absorb the nutrients from the food and deposit them into the blood stream to be taken all around the body.

The blood when passing through the lungs also absorbs oxygen that we have inhaled.

So the blood carries the nutrients and the oxygen essential for the cells in our body to break down the nutrients into packets of energy.

Thus the cells of our body get nutrients and oxygen from blood, break down the nutrients into energy and Life is Sustained!!!

But like any other mechanism in this universe, every step produces a byproduct in form of waste.

The food post-digestion in excreted form the intestines in form of stool.

Impurities in our blood are separated in our kidneys and excreted in form of urine.

The impurities/toxins created at the cellular level are in two forms, liquid and volatile.

The liquid toxins are put out by our skin in form of sweat. (You will be surprised to know that our skin is the largest excretory organ in our body)

The volatile toxins (which are most harmful) are thrown out in form of toxic gases using our lungs, when we BREATHE OUT!!!

Pranayama plays a pivotal role here in ridding our bodies of these harmful toxins.

It supplies our lungs and hence our blood with abundant supply of fresh oxygen.

It boosts our immune system.

It is amazingly effective in calming down your mind.

It helps in improving our memory, virility and strengthens our neurological system.

There are many other Pranayama techniques which can be used for multiple other purposes.

(I will tell you everything about those techniques, don't worry :))

There are 7 Pranayama techniques which are widely known and practiced.

Yet, there are many more techniques (almost 50+ that I came across during my study of Pranayama techiques) which are not easily available to the common public,

but have to be actively searched for in various scriptures and Upanishads, which work wonders and are nearly miraculous in their effectiveness.

Starting with the most commonly known ones, I have compiled the most effective and beneficial 14 of those breathing techniques in this book for you.

Let's get down to business...

Some Important Terminologies

Here are some terminologies you'll come across in this book:

Breathing Terminologies-

Purak-

To inhale in to the full capacity of your lungs. Also, when you inhale don't expand your stomach instead fill all the air in your chest.

Kumbhak-

('Kumbh' means a pot or a round utensil) To hold the inhaled air in your lungs.

Rechak-

To exhale every ounce of air out of your lungs.

Bandh or Lock terminologies-

Jalandhar Bandh-

To close your wind pipe by pressing your chin against the base of your neck.

Uddiyan Bandh-

To contract your abdomen and try to suck in your stomach so that it will touch your spine.

Mula Bandh-

To pull in your anal muscles. (it is as if you have to go to the toilet but are not able to find one nearby and you have to hold it in.)

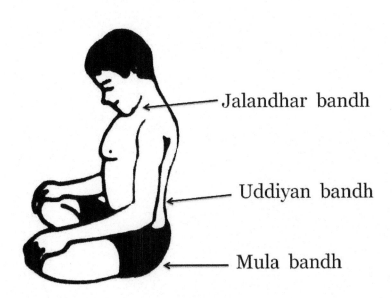

Jalandhar bandh

Uddiyan bandh

Mula bandh

Pranayama

Seating Position for performing Pranayama

Most of the Pranayama are to be performed while sitting in *'Sukhasan'* position.

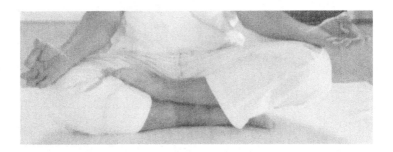

Sukhasan (the Simple Sitting Pose)

-Sit on the mat with your legs stretched in front.

-Fold the right leg and tug in below the left thigh.

-Then, fold the left leg and tug it between the right thigh and calf.

-Sit straight with an erect spine.

(It is how we generally sit on the floor and fold our legs.)

Pranayama #1

Bhastrika Pranayama/ Bellow Breath

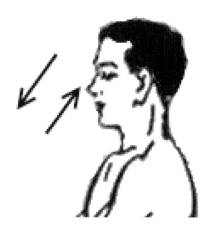

Method:

Sit in Sukhasan and form the dnyanamudra with your hands and place them on your knees with your palms facing upwards.

('Dnyanamudra' is formed when you join the tips of your index finger and your thumb while keeping your other fingers outstretched.)

Close your eyes.

Inhale to your full capacity; hold the breath in for a couple of seconds and then exhale slowly.

When you inhale, fill the air into your lungs and expand your chest while inhaling and it will press your diaphragm down;

Do not expand your stomach while inhaling.

Concentrate completely on your breathing and pay attention to how you feel with every breath you take.

Visualize, every breath nourishing all the parts of your body.

Duration:

Perform this Pranayama for at least 3 minutes.

Uses:

-This is a nourishing exercise and it enhances your digestive capabilities and creates heat in the body.

-It helps in burning the excess fat.

-It helps in reducing the amount of phlegm.

-It is very effective in cases of Asthma.

-It strengthens your Lungs.

-It helps in purifying blood and facilitates efficient blood circulation.

Pranayama #2

Kapaalbhati Pranayama/Pranayama for forehead cleanse

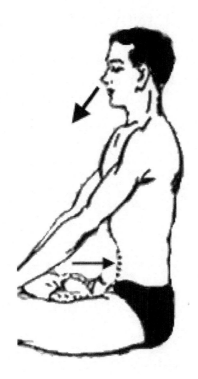

Method:

Sit in Sukhasan and form the dnyanamudra with your hands and place them on your knees with your palms facing upwards.

Close your eyes.

Then, exhale quickly in a single stroke/movement. Your lungs will contract in that moment and your stomach will be sucked in.

Don't inhale purposefully; once you exhale rapidly inhaling will happen as a reflex.

Keep repeating the exhaling action and with every breath that comes out visualize every impurity within, every toxic matter and each negative thought is being thrown out of your body.

Caution:

- People suffering from back pain and waist pain should perform the exhaling motion a bit slowly.

- People suffering with Heart diseases should perform the exhaling motion slowly.

- Pregnant women should NOT practice this Pranayama.

Duration:

Practice this Pranayama for 4-5 minutes in the start, but with regular practice gradually increase the duration to 12-15 minutes. (If at the start you feel tired after a few minutes, stop for a few seconds and then continue again.)

Uses:

You will be amazed with the benefits of this Pranayama:

-It is very helpful in burning excess fat.

-It is very helpful in regulating your blood sugar levels and thus keeps diabetes in check.

-It is found to be very effective in clearing heart blockages in people suffering from arteriosclerosis. (but please perform the exhaling motion slowly)

-It maintains the health of your liver.

-It helps in getting rid of constipation.

-It is even observed that a regular practice of this Pranayama cures Hepatitis.

-It reduces the amount of phlegm in your body and is also very helpful for patients suffering from Asthma.

-It is very helpful for people suffering from pollen and dust allergies.

-It is observed that a regular practice of this Pranayama reduces the size of Tumors and cysts in the body. (There have been many cases where patients have reported that their tumors have completely dissolved due to a regular and disciplined practice of this Pranayama.)

-In women it is found to cure any uterine ailments.

-It is even found to be extremely effective in curing skin diseases.

-It is very effective in curing diseases of the throat.

-It brings a peculiar glow to the aura of the practitioner.

Pranayama #3

Bahya Pranayama/Exterior Pranayama

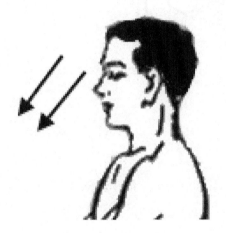

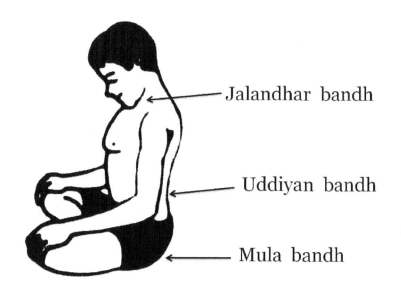

Jalandhar bandh

Uddiyan bandh

Mula bandh

Method:

Sit in Sukhasan and form the dnyanamudra with your hands and place them on your knees with your palms facing upwards.

Close your eyes.

Inhale to your full capacity; hold the breath in for a couple of seconds and then exhale with a bit of force such that you are trying to empty your lungs rapidly. (It will make a screeching sound at the end of your exhalation)

After complete exhalation implement the following 3 blocks-

Perform the *'Muladharbandh'* (Pull in your anal muscles as if you are trying to hold in your bowels).

Perform the *'Uddiyanbandh'* (Pull in your stomach, as if you are trying to touch your stomach to the Spine).

Perform the 'Jalandharbandh' (Press your chin on your throat and look straight down).

Don't inhale for a few seconds and then remove all the three blocks mentioned above and slowly inhale to your full capacity.

Caution:

-People suffering from heart problems **should not** practice this Pranayama.

-People suffering from Cervical problems and Spondilitis should not implement the Jalandharbandh (3rd block)

Duration:

No specific duration, but perform this Pranayama only 3-4 times.

Uses:

-It strengthens your stomach.

-It enhances your digestive capabilities.

-It is very helpful for curing hernia.

- It maintains the health of your thyroid.

-It strengthens your lungs.

-Its most effective application is that it amplifies the effects of Kapaalbhati Pranayama.

Pranayama #4

Suryabhedan Pranayama/Pranayama of the Sun

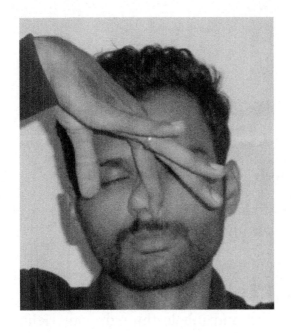

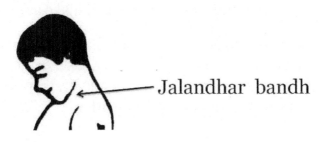

Jalandhar bandh

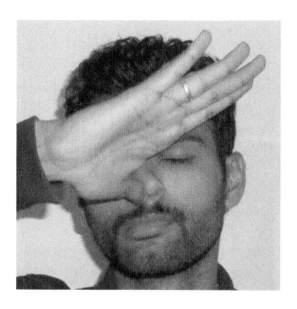

Method:

Sit in Sukhasan and keep your left hand on your left knee with your palm facing down.

Close your eyes.

Close your left nostril with the index finger of your right hand and inhale through your right nostril untill your lungs are full. (Inhale with a bit of force, so that the air gushing in will make a sound)

Once your lungs are full, hold the air in and perform the 'Jalandharbandh' [Neck Lock](Press your chin on your throat and look straight down) as long as you can hold your breath in.

Close your right nostril with the thumb of your right hand, remove the neck lock and exhale through your left nostril and apply enough force that your exhaling too will make a sound.

This is one round of Suryabhedan Pranayama.

Duration:

Initially do only 2-3 rounds or repetitions of this Pranaym. Increase it gradually to 10-12 rounds in one session.

Uses:

-Regular practice of this Pranayama reduces the amount of cough and phlegm in your body.

-It is very helpful in removing toxic gases from your body.

-It generates heat within one's body.

-It helps in blood purification.

-It enhances one's digestive capabilities.

Pranayama #5

Anulobh-Vilobh Pranayama/
Pranayama of complete Detox

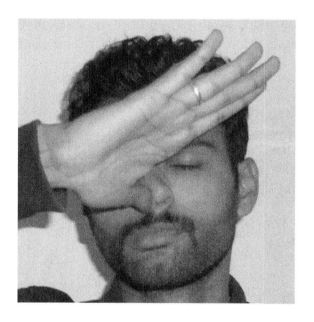

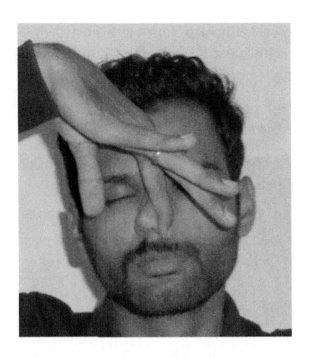

Method:

Sit in Sukhasan and form the dnyanamudra with your left hand and place it on your left knee with your palms facing upwards.

Close your eyes.

Close your right nostril with the thumb of your right hand and inhale through your left nostril till your lungs are full.

Then close your left nostril with the ring and middle finger of your right hand and exhale through your right nostril.

Inhale back through your right nostril then close your right nostril with the thumb and exhale through your left nostril,

Then inhale back through your left nostril and exhale through your right nostril.

Pay attention to it that, you inhale through the same nostril that you have used to exhale.

And see to it that there is no hurry while doing this Pranayama. Be comfortable, calm and perform it slowly.

Duration:

At first perform it for 3-4 minutes and then with practice, gradually increase the time to 12-15 minutes.

Uses:

-It is the most effective detox exercise.

-It throws out all the toxins out of the body through your breath.

-It is an excellent cure for hypertension.

-It is very helpful in curing ear disorders.

-When performed regularly, it prevents the occurrence of cancer.

-It is found to be helpful in curing leukoderma.

-It is very helpful in curing bronchitis.

Pranayama #6

Bhramari Pranayama/Pranayama of the Hornet

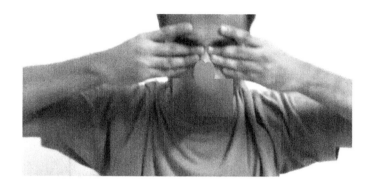

Method:

Sit in Sukhasan.

Close your eyes.

Then close your ears with your thumbs, place your index fingers on your forehead, and place the remaining three fingers on your eyes and press the ridge between your eyes slightly with your middle finger.

Inhale to your full capacity; hold the breath in for a couple of seconds.

Then keeping your mouth closed, exhale slowly while making the 'Aum' sound (Om Chant).

(This step creates a sound similar to the buzzing of a hornet's wings hence the name.)

Duration:

No specific duration. Repeat it for at least 2-3 times.

Uses:

-This Pranayama is extremely essential for maintaining the health of your throat and thyroid.

-It cures any hoarseness of voice caused by any illness.

-Regular practice of this Pranayama increases your concentration and also calms your mind.

-You'll feel a soothing peace and calmness when you perform this Pranayama regularly.

Pranayama #7

Udgith Pranayama/Pranayama of resounding Aum

Method:

Sit in Sukhasan and form the dnyanamudra with your hands and place them on your knees with your palms facing upwards.

Close your eyes.

Inhale to your full capacity; hold the breath in for a couple of seconds and then exhale through the chant of 'Aum'.

Listen to this chant as it fills your surroundings with the sound of cosmic vibrations.

Duration:

Repeat it for 3-4 times.

Uses:

-This Pranayama is very effective in curing any disorders of the throat, lungs and upper chest.

-It maintains a proper blood circulation and also helps in purifying your blood.

Pranayama #8

Detox Breath I

Method:

Stand up without slouching and with your back straight.

Keep a space of 10-12 inches between your feet.

See to it that your body weight is equally distributed on both your feet.

Put out your chest, keep your neck straight and slightly pull down your chin.

Keep your hands at your sides with your palms touching your thighs.

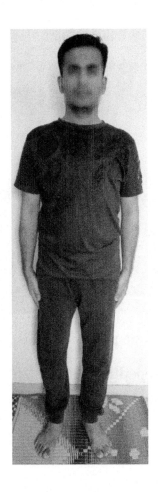

Now, slowly but steadily take in a deep breath.

First fill in your chest with air, once the chest is full then, fill the air in your belly.

Hold the air in for as long as you comfortably can.

Then open your mouth and rapidly exhale through your mouth by contracting your stomach but keeping your chest rigid.

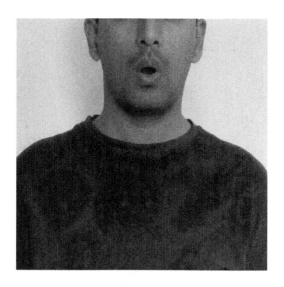

This completes one practice of this Pranayama.

Perform 8-10 repetitions.

Take a rest of 1-2 min. before doing anything else.

Uses:

-This Pranayama is especially effective in pushing the volatile toxins from the lungs and the stomach out of the body

-Also, this breath rejuvenates the organs in the chest cavity and neck.

Pranayama #9

Lung Strengthening Breath I

Method:

Stand up without slouching and with your back straight.

Keep a space of 10-12 inches between your feet.

See to it that your body weight is equally distributed on both your feet.

Put out your chest, keep your neck straight and slightly pull down your chin.

Keep your hands at chest height, with your palms facing you.

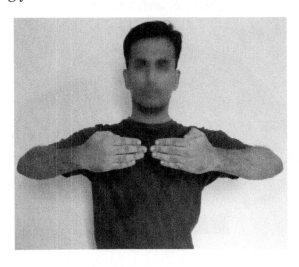

Now, slowly but steadily take in a deep breath.

As you are breathing in, initiating at the base of your collar bone, start to firmly pat down your chest cavity till you reach your abdomen.

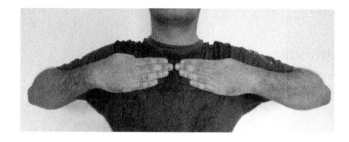

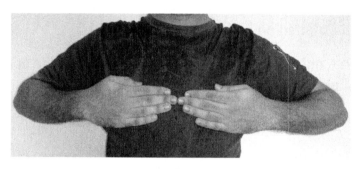

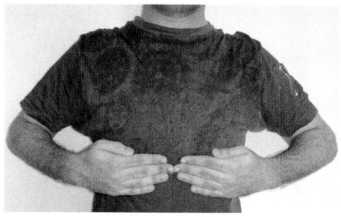

Fill in your lungs to their full capacity.

Once your lungs are full, start to lightly massage your chest in vertical motions.

Continue massaging your chest for as long as you could hold your breath in.

Then exhale slowly and steadily with your hands by your side.

This completes one practice of this Pranayama.

Perform 7-8 repetitions.

Take a rest of 1 or 2 min. before doing anything else.

Uses:

-This Pranayama is very effective in curing any disorders of the lungs and upper chest.

-It maintains proper blood circulation around your chest and is helpful in improving blood flow in the capillaries of the lungs.

Pranayama #10

Lung Strengthening Breath II

Method:

Stand up without slouching and with your back straight.

Keep your feet shoulder length apart.

See to it that your body weight is equally distributed on both your feet.

Put out your chest, keep your neck straight.

Put your hands under your respective armpits with your fingers in the front and thumb at the back.

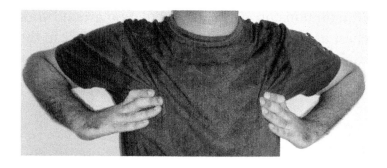

Now, slowly but steadily take in a deep breath.

Fill in your lungs to their full capacity.

Now hold in your breath for as long as you comfortably can.

Then when you have to exhale, press your ribcage from the sides and start slowly exhaling.

The exhaling motion should be done in installments. Press & exhale – stop – press & exhale – stop again, till you have completely exhaled.

This completes one practice of this Pranayama.

Perform 5 repetitions.

Uses:

-This Pranayama is very effective in increasing your lung capacity.

-It also helps in purifying your blood and rejuvenating the cells and tissues of the inner lining of your lungs.

Pranayama #11

Quick Rejuvenating Breath

Method:

Stand up without slouching and with your back straight.

Keep your feet shoulder length apart.

See to it that your body weight is equally distributed on both your feet.

Put out your chest, keep your neck straight.

Put your hands under your respective armpits with your fingers in the front and thumb at the back.

Then slide your hand down where the ribcage ends and the abdomen begins.

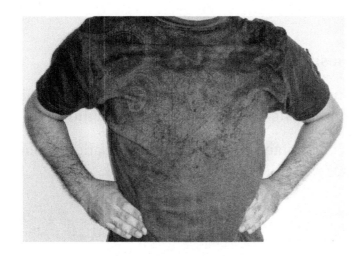

Now, slowly but steadily take in a deep breath.

Fill in your lungs to their full capacity.

Now hold in your breath for as long as you comfortably can.

Then when you have to exhale, press the end of your ribcage from the sides and start slowly exhaling.

The exhaling motion should be done in installments. Press & exhale – stop – press & exhale – stop again, till you have completely exhaled.

This completes one practice of this Pranayama.

Perform 5-7 repetitions.

Take a rest of 3-4 min. before doing anything else.

Uses:

-This breath is very effective in providing quick rejuvenation and alertness to the practitioner.

- It maintains proper blood circulation around your chest and the abdominal organs.

Pranayama #12

Inspiring Breath I

Method:

Stand up without slouching and with your back straight.

Keep a space of 10-12 inches between your feet.

See to it that your body weight is equally distributed on both your feet.

Put out your chest, keep your neck straight and slightly pull down your chin.

Keep your hands at your sides with your palms touching your thighs.

Concentrate your eyes at the tip of your nose and bring a smile on your face. (You have to continuously maintain a smile on your face while performing this Pranayama.)

Now, slowly but steadily take in a deep breath.

As you are breathing in, lift up your toes in the air.

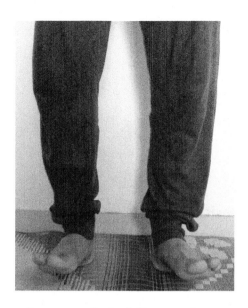

Fill in your lungs to their full capacity.

Once your inhalation is complete, stand on your toes and lift up your heels in the air.

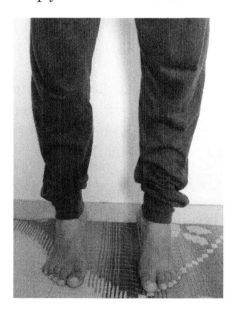

Remain in this position till you are holding in your breath for 8-10 seconds.

Then slowly exhaling return back to you initial standing position.

This completes one practice of this Pranayama.

Perform 10-12 repetitions.

Take a rest of 2 min. before doing anything else.

Uses:

-This breathing technique, busts your stress, calms you down and fills the practitioner with vigor to do something new.

Pranayama #13

Inspiring Breath II

Method:

Stand up without slouching and with your back straight.

Keep a space of 10-12 inches between your feet.

See to it that your body weight is equally distributed on both your feet.

Put out your chest, keep your neck straight and slightly pull down your chin.

Keep your hands at your sides with your palms touching your thighs.

Now, slowly but steadily take in a deep breath.

As you are breathing in, lift up your hands slowly over your head. Let your palms touch each other and then press them together as firmly as you can without bending your hands at the elbows. This will send vibrations down hands and into your shoulders and unto your upper chest.

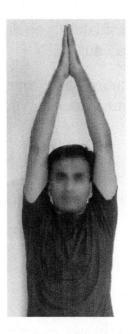

Once your inhalation is complete, stop pressing your palms together and stand on your toes and lift up your heels in the air.

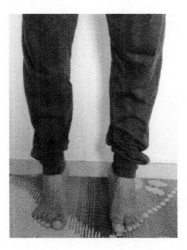

Remain in this position till you are holding in your breath for 8-10 seconds.

Then slowly exhaling take your hands down to your side and return back to you initial standing position.

This completes one practice of this Pranayama.

Perform 5-7 repetitions.

Take a rest of 2 min. before doing anything else.

Uses:

-This Pranayama brings a unique serenity and calmness to the practitioner.

-It also maintains proper blood circulation in the limbs.

Pranayama #14

Heart Strengthening Breath

Method:

Stand up without slouching and with your back straight.

Keep a space of 10-12 inches between your feet.

See to it that your body weight is equally distributed on both your feet.

Put out your chest, keep your neck straight and look straight ahead.

Raise your hands in front of you to shoulder height, with your palms facing each other.

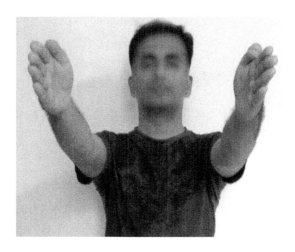

Now, slowly but steadily take in a deep breath.

As you are breathing in, move your hands to your sides and then to back as much as you can. (all the while keeping them parallel to the ground)

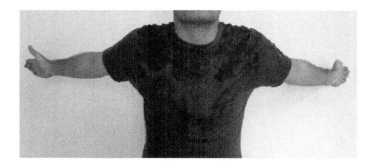

Once your inhalation is complete, remain in this position till you are holding in your breath for 12-15 seconds.

Then slowly exhaling take your hands back to you initial standing position.

This completes one practice of this Pranayama.

Perform 8-10 repetitions.

Take a rest of 1-2 min. before doing anything else.

Uses:

-This Pranayama is very effective in strengthening our heart muscles and your lungs.

-It maintains a proper blood circulation and also helps in purifying your blood.

What's Next?

This Book has laid the foundation for you to start a routine practice of Pranayama.

Now the ball is in your court.

You can keep living as it is, or decide to use this new-found knowledge for your benefit and the well-being of your loved ones too.

All you need is a mat to sit on and a few minutes for yourself in the morning.

That is all it takes.

Remember, Easy Does It!!!

Thank You!!

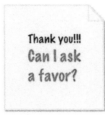

Thank you so much for reading my book. I hope you really liked it.

As you probably know, many people look at the reviews on Amazon before they decide to purchase a book.

If you liked the book, please take a minute to leave a review with your feedback.

60 seconds is all I'm asking for, and it would mean a lot to me.

Thank You so much.

All the best,

Advait

BOOK EXCERPT: "Mudras for Beginners"

Pranayama

'Mudras for Beginners'

Your Ultimate Beginners Guide to using Simple Hand Gestures for Everlasting Health, Rapid Weight Loss and Easy Self Healing

by

Advait

What are Mudras?

According to the Vedic culture of ancient India, our entire world is made of 'the five elements' called as *The Panch-Maha-Bhuta's*. The five elements being **Earth**, **Water**, **Fire**, **Wind** and **Space/Vacuum**. They are also called the earth element, water element, fire element, wind element and space element.

These five elements constitute the human body – the nutrients from the soil (earth) are absorbed by the plants which we consume (thus we survive on the earth element), the blood flowing through own veins represents the water element, the body heat represents the fire element, the oxygen we inhale and the carbon dioxide we exhale represents the wind element and the sinuses we have in our nose and skull represent the space element.

As long as these five elements in our body are balanced and maintain appropriate levels we remain healthy. An imbalance of these elements in the human body leads to a deteriorated health and diseases.

Now understand this, the command and control center of all these five elements lies in our fingers. So literally, our health lies at our fingertips.

The Mudra healing method that I am going to teach you depends on our fingers.

To understand this, we should first know the finger-element relationship:

Thumb – Fire element.

Index finger – Air element.

Middle finger – Space/Vacuum element.

Third finger – Earth element.

Small finger – Water element.

This image will give you a better understanding of the concept:

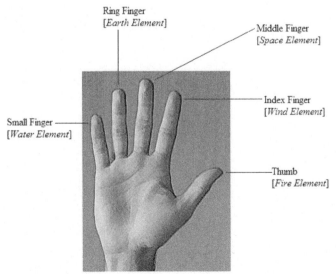

When the fingers are brought together in a specific pattern and are touched to each other, or slightly pressed against each other, the formation is called as a 'Mudra'.

When the five fingers are touched and pressed in a peculiar way to form a Mudra, it affects the levels of the five elements in our body, thus balancing those elements and inducing good health.

P.S. The Mudra Healing Methods aren't just theory or wordplay; these are healing methods from the ancient Indian Vedic culture, proven and tested over ages.

How Do These Mudras Work?

To understand how the Mudras work, we first need to know the 'Prakriti' concept of Ayurveda.

Prakriti *(The Basic Bodily Constitution)*

According to Ayurveda, every person is constituted of the Three Dosha's - The *Vata* Dosha, The *Pitta* Dosha and The *Kapha* Dosha.

And, any one of the three Dosha's is most dominant among them, which determines the basic or primary constitution or *Prakriti* of an individual.

The core concept of Ayurvedic medicine is that, the five fundamental elements integrate into physical form as the three *Doshas* and health exists when there is a balance between the three fundamental bodily *Doshas* known as: *Vata, Pitta* and *Kapha*.

The physical volume of a human being is mainly composed of *Kapha,* the chemical processes and reactions taking place in the body are due to the manifestation of *Pitta*, and the bodily movements and activities are attributed to *Vata*.

For an individual to remain healthy, these three basic substances (*doshas*) must be in equilibrium. Any kind of disequilibrium of these *doshas* will cause disintegration of the body which leads to disease.

When we consume food, it is digested and nutrients (*Saara*) and waste/excreta (*Mala*) are produced. The nutrients nourish the seven bodily tissues (*SaptaDhatu's*) and the waste is thrown out of the body through sweat, urine, feces, nasal discharge, eye discharge etc., while this is happening the three doshas move from one part of the body to another part and induce sound health, resistance to disease and physical strength in an individual. But, if the *doshas* are excited or vitiated they produce disease in the body.

Vata

Vata is the air principle necessary to mobilize the function of the nervous system.

The main functions of *Vata* are to give motion to the body, conduction of impulses from sensory organs, separation of nutrient and waste from food, secretion of urine and semen.

In healthy condition it performs all the physiological functions in the body, it is responsible for speech & hearing, it regulates the normal circulation in the body and it is also responsible for formation and development of foetus in intra-uterine stage.

When excited or vitiated, it produces psychosomatic disorder, causes weight loss, loss of physical strength and it may cause congenital deformities.

Pitta

Pitta is the fire principle which uses bile to direct digestion and hence metabolism into the venous system.

The endocrine functions in the body and other biological activities in the human body are caused by *Pitta*. It is the by-product of human blood (Rakta).

Pitta is homologous of blood and both are situated/originate in spleen and liver.

Pitta can be physically observed, it is a yellow coloured viscous liquid, it has a fleshy and unpleasant smell and it feels hot when touched.

Pitta provides volume and colour to blood, induces proper digestion, proper vision. It is responsible for body heat, appetite, thirst, complexion and intelligence.

Kapha

Kapha is the water principle which relates to mucous, lubrication and the carrier of nutrients into the arterial system.

When compared to *Vata* and *Pitta*, *Kapha* is the most stable of the three doshas and it is mainly composed of water. It is responsible for formation of bodily structures.

It is white in colour, thick, viscous, slimy and soft to touch. The body owes its softness, smoothness, moisture and coolness to *Kapha*.

The *Kapha* joints together various structures of the body and the joints. It promotes healing, immunity and tissue-building within the body. *Kapha* provides stability, physical strength and sturdiness to one's body.

The Dosha - Element - Finger Relationship

Remember the finger-element relationship image I showed you earlier? That comes into play now...

Vata Dosha – Air Element + Space/vacuum Element

Thus the levels of 'Vata' in your body can be very easily manipulated/changed/regulated by using your index finger, middle finger and Thumb.

Pitta Dosha – Fire Element + Water Element

The levels of 'Pitta' in your body can be regulated by using your small finger and Thumb.

Kapha Dosha – Water Element + Earth Element

The levels of 'Kapha' in your body can be regulated by using your small finger and ring finger.

The Mudra healing technique is based on understanding the imbalances in your dosha's which are the underlying cause of your disease and then regulating and balancing your dosha's through simple hand gestures and curing you without any external medication.

Fingers – Control Knobs of Your Health

Mudras are broadly classified into two types;

#1 (असंयुक्त) *Asanyunkt Mudra* – Mudra performed on each hand individually, e.g. Dnyanmudra.

#2 (संयुक्त) *Sanyukt Mudra* – Mudra performed by using both the hands, e.g. Dhenumudra.

But, this is the external physical aspect of these Mudras, let's now see how our fingers act as 3 Mode control knobs for inducing good health.

Here's the' Element – Finger' relationship again;

Thumb – Fire element.

Index finger – Air element.

Middle finger – Space/Vacuum element.

Third finger – Earth element.

Small finger – Water element.

Mode I-

Balancing the Element: when the tip of a finger is touched to the tip of the thumb and pressed slightly, it results in regulating the level of the element associated with that finger in harmony with the other elements.

e.g. In *Dnyanmudra* the tip of the index finger and thumb are touched together, this results in a regulation and balancing of air element in the human body.

Mode II-

Enhancing the Element: When the tip of the thumb is touched to the base of a finger and pressed slightly, it results in increasing the level of the element associated with that finger.

e.g. In *Avaahanmudra* the tip of the thumb is touched to the base of the small finger, this results in an increase in the water element of the body, thus curing you of any disease related to deficiency of water element.

Mode III-

Suppressing the Element: When a finger is curled down and the nail of that finger is covered by the tip of the thumb or when the tip of the finger touches the base of the thumb and the thumb covers over the back of the finger, it results in reducing the level of the element associated with that finger.

e.g. In *Vaayumudra* the tip of the index finger touches the base of the thumb and the thumb cover over the back of the index finger, this results in a reduction in the air element of the body, thus curing you of any disease related to an increase in air element.

Can I perform these Mudras?

Yes!!! Anyone and everyone can perform these simple hand gestures and benefit from them.

Men-Women, Young-Old, Kids... anyone can perform these Mudras.

There are no exceptions but just precautions –

a) There are certain Mudras which are off limits for pregnant women. (Which I have mentioned specifically as a note under the description of those Mudras).

b) People suffering with arthritis will find it difficult to perform these mudras initially and for longer period of time, but they should nevertheless attempt to practice these mudras for a shorter period of time, till they feel comfortable doing them. With time you will see that the regular practice of these mudras you will be able to perform these mudras for their full prescribed time.

When and for How long can I perform these Mudras?

When-

That is the beauty of Mudra healing, You Can Practice These Mudras Anyplace-Anytime.

- while travelling/commuting
- while watching TV, sitting on your favorite couch
- while reading your favorite book or newspaper or magazine
- while chatting with your friends and family
- while walking your dog
- while you are waiting for someone
- while Meditating

How Long-

For the basic beginner Mudras there is no specific time limit, but for best results these Mudras should be practiced for at least 35-40 minutes at a stretch.

[Start by practicing these Mudras for 10 minutes each and then gradually increase the time limit till you reach your 40 minutes target.]

For other complex Mudras the time limit varies depending upon the ailment that we are curing and I have duly specified the essential time limit in such cases.

What are the other precautions I should take?

There are no other precautions to be taken, just see to it that you are completely relaxed and are breathing normally when you perform these Mudras.

Don't forget to do some warm up exercises before practicing the Mudras to avoid sore hands afterwards.

Warm-Up exercises for preparing your Hands

Before practicing these Mudras it is best to do some warm up exercises for your palms, to avoid any further inconvenience or any possible discomfort.

Warm up-

Step I: make a fist on both your palms, hold for a few seconds and then release the fist and extend the fingers outwards. Repeat 8-10 times.

Step II: Clap lightly for 15-20 seconds without stopping. Repeat 2-3 times.

Step III: Rub your palms together for around 40-45 seconds so that they become warm.

Now, you are all set to start practicing these Mudras.

11 Basic Mudras for Beginners

Pranayama

Attention!!!

Read this First

For the better understanding of the reader, a detail image/sketch has been provided for every mudra along with the method to perform it, but the image given is only of the right hand performing the Mudra.

The Mudras shown in this book are to be performed simultaneously on both your hands for the Mudras to have the maximum healing effect, only exception being the Mudras requiring both your hands to form a Mudra.

Mudra #1

Dnyanamudra / Mudra of Wisdom

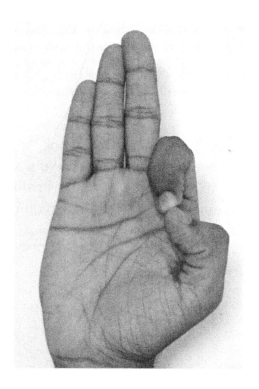

Method:

Sit in a comfortable position.

Your head, neck and spine should be in straight alignment.

Now, touch the tip of your thumb with the tip of your index finger and press slightly.

Keep all the other fingers straight as shown in the image.

(Thumb represents the fire element while the index finger represents the wind element, this mudra brings together the fire and wind elements.)

Duration:

No time limit for this Mudra and it can be done at any time you wish.

Uses:

Helps in attaining a peaceful mind.

Increases concentration.

Sharpens your brain thus increasing intelligence.

Anxiety, Anger and Laziness just disappear when you perform this Mudra.

Most importantly, this Mudra regulates the hormonal secretion by Pituitary and Pineal glands.

This Mudra is extensively used in curing Insomnia.

In cases of Migraine, Dnyanamudra done together with Praanamudra have proved to be very helpful.

This Mudra should be practiced frequently and for longer durations by anyone who is facing any kind of psychological disorders.

Mudra #2

Akashmudra / Mudra of Sky

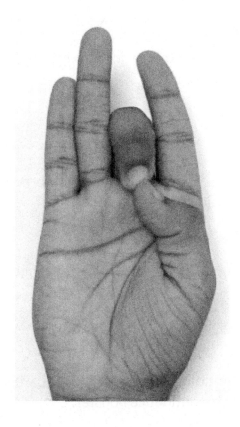

Method:

Touch the tip of your thumb with the tip of your middle finger.

Keep all the other fingers straight as shown in the image.

(here we bring the fire element and the space element together.)

Duration:

No time limit for this Mudra and it can be done at any time you wish.

Uses:

This Mudra is especially useful for people with Heart Disorders.

This Mudra strengthens your Heart.

Performing this Mudra regularly strengthens your bones.

In cases of a locked jaw, this mudra works as a charm.

On an emotional level, this Mudra works as an amazing self-confidence booster.

It helps in strengthening your teeth.

This Mudra should be regularly performed by people with Heart disorders and Bone disorders.

Mudra #3

Prithvimudra / Mudra of Earth

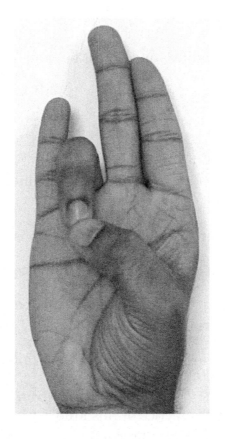

Method:

Touch the tip of your thumb with the tip of your ring finger and press slightly.

Keep all the other fingers straight as shown in the image.

(here we bring the fire element and the earth element together.)

Duration:

15 to 35 minutes, and it can be done at any time you wish.

Uses:

Performing this Mudra regularly reduces physical weakness.

If you want to gain weight this Mudra is for you.

This Mudra is helpful in improving digestion.

After doing this Mudra you will feel and look extremely fresh.

If you are feeling down, this Mudra will elevate your mood.

With regular practice of this Mudra you will notice a peculiar glow of your skin.

This Mudra is also believed to channel in positive energy into your body from the earth.

Mudra #4

Varunmudra / Mudra of Rain God

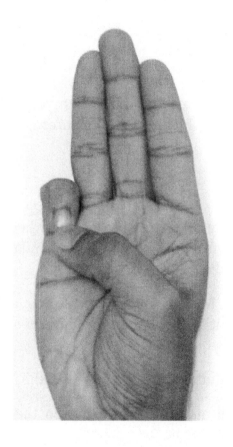

Method:

Touch the tip of your thumb with the tip of your small finger (pinkie finger) and press slightly.

Keep all the other fingers straight as shown in the image.

(here we bring the fire element and the water element together, which means we are burning away all the contamination and internal debris induced by the water element.)

Duration:

15 to 35 minutes and only when you suffer from the ailments which this Mudra cures.

Uses:

This Mudra is extremely useful when you are suffering from Diarrhea and similar Gastro-intestinal disorders.

Since this Mudra balances the water element in our body, it's a very helpful Mudra in any type of Skin disease.

Also this Mudra reduces swelling of the intestine.

If you feel any kind of itching on the skin, this Mudra will cure it.

This Mudra helps in relieving strained Muscles.

This Mudra is also called as 'Preserver of Youth'.

Mudra #5

Vaayumudra / Mudra of Air

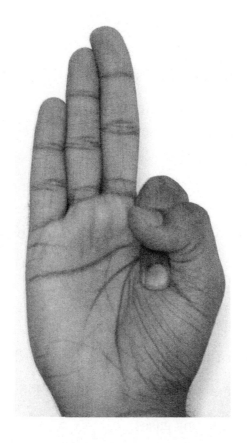

Method:

Touch the base of your thumb with the tip of your index finger as shown in the image.

Advait

Slightly press your thumb on the bent index finger.

Keep all the other fingers straight as shown in the image.

(here the fire element presses the wind element)

Duration:

For 15 minutes, 3 times a day.

The duration can be increased to 30 - 35 minutes depending upon the seriousness of the ailment.

Uses:

This Mudra helps in reducing the increased wind element.

Helps in trembling and shivers.

Helps in arthritis and joint pains.

This Mudra strengthens your Spinal cord.

Helps in maintaining a proper Blood Flow.

Helps in reducing gases.

On an emotional level, this Mudra increases concentration.

Note:

Performing a *'Pranamudra'* after the *'Vaayumudra'* enhances its effects.

---------- **End of Excerpt** ----------

If you wish to read the entire book, It is available for FREE on Amazon.

Visit the link below the image.

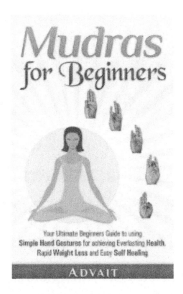

Other books on Mudras by Advait

P.S. All my books are enrolled in the 'Kindle Unlimited Program' you can read all of my books for free through **'Kindle Unlimited'.**

Mudras for Awakening Chakras: 19 Simple Hand Gestures for Awakening & Balancing Your Chakras

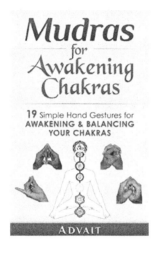

http://www.amazon.com/dp/B00P82COAY

[#1 Bestseller in 'Yoga']

[#1 Bestseller in 'Chakras']

Pranayama

Mudras for Weight Loss: 21 Simple Hand Gestures for Effortless Weight Loss

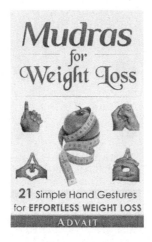

http://www.amazon.com/dp/B00P3ZPSEK

Mudras for Spiritual Healing: 21 Simple Hand Gestures for Ultimate Spiritual Healing & Awakening

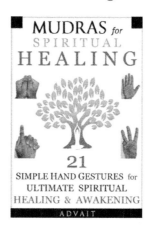

http://www.amazon.com/dp/B00PFYZLQO

Mudras for Women: 25 Simple Hand Gestures every Woman should know for attaining a healthy body, beautiful skin, supercharged sex drive and enhanced vitality

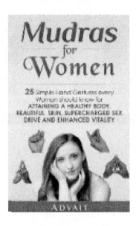

Mudras: 25 Ultimate techniques for Self Healing

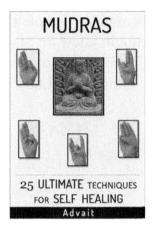

http://www.amazon.com/dp/B00MMPB5CI

Mudras for Anxiety: 25 Simple Hand Gestures for Curing Your Anxiety

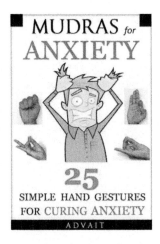

http://www.amazon.com/dp/B00PF011IU

Mudras for Sex: 25 Simple Hand Gestures for
Extreme Erotic Pleasure & Sexual Vitality

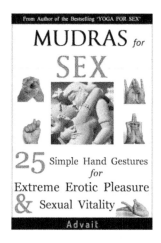

http://www.amazon.com/dp/B00OJR1DRY

Pranayama

Mudras for a Strong Heart: 21 Simple Hand
Gestures for Preventing, Curing & Reversing Heart
Disease

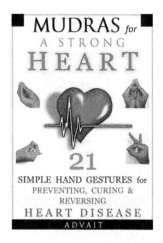

http://www.amazon.com/dp/B00PFRLGTM

Mudras for Stress Management: 21 Simple Hand
Gestures for a Stress Free Life

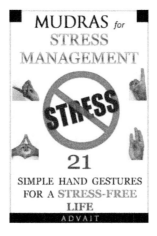

http://amazon.com/dp/B00PFTJ6OC

Mudras for Memory Improvement: 25 Simple
Hand Gestures for Ultimate Memory
Improvement

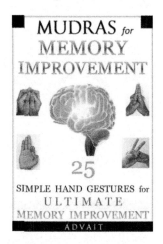

http://www.amazon.com/dp/B00PFSP8TK

Mudras for Curing Cancer: 21 Simple Hand
Gestures for Preventing & Curing Cancer

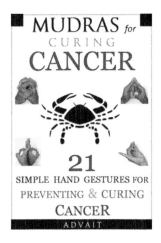

http://www.amazon.com/dp/B00PFO199M

Pranayama

Notes

<u>Notes</u>

<u>Notes</u>

<u>Notes</u>

<u>Notes</u>

Printed in Great Britain
by Amazon

18781058R00068